High Fiber Foods

Chapter List:

The Power of Fiber: An Introduction to a Healthier You
Whole Grains: The Foundation of a High-Fiber Diet
The Benefits of Legumes: Fueling Your Body with Fiber
The Green Revolution: Exploring Fiber-Rich Vegetables
Fruity Delights: How Fiber-Packed Fruits Boost Your Well-being

The Nutty Way: Nurturing Your Body with Fiber-Rich Nuts and Seeds
Fantastic Fiber: Unveiling the Magic of Fiber Supplements
Fiber and Digestion: Enhancing Gut Health and Relieving Digestive Issues
Fiber and Weight Management: The Key to Shedding Pounds Naturally
Fiber and Heart Health: Protecting Your Most Vital Organ
Fiber and Diabetes: Regulating Blood Sugar Levels Naturally
Fiber and Detoxification: Cleansing Your Body from Within
Fiber for Healthy Skin: Unveiling the Beauty Benefits of Fiber
Fiber and Mental Health: Nurturing Your Mind through Proper Nutrition
Practical Tips for Incorporating Fiber into Your Daily Routine

Book Introduction:

In a world where fast food and processed meals dominate our plates, it's no wonder that our bodies are yearning for proper nutrition. The High Fiber diet is here to revolutionize the way we eat and pave the path to a healthier and more fulfilling life. This book, "High Fiber: Nourishing Your Body, Enriching Your Life," will serve as your guide to understanding the importance of fiber and how it can transform your well-being.

Through the pages of this book, you will embark on a journey of discovery, uncovering the secrets behind the power of fiber and its immense benefits for your body and mind. From the wonders of whole grains and legumes to the abundant goodness found in vegetables, fruits, nuts, and seeds, each chapter will delve into the wonders of these high-fiber foods and provide you with valuable insights into their impact on your overall health.

But this book is not merely a collection of facts and figures. It is a celebration of the emotional connection we have with food and the profound impact it can have on our lives. With an emphasis on an emotional tone, "High Fiber: Nourishing Your Body, Enriching Your Life" will ignite a passion within you to prioritize your well-being and embark on a transformative journey toward a healthier lifestyle.

So, get ready to indulge your senses and feed your soul as you dive into the world of high-fiber foods. Let the chapters that follow be your guiding light, illuminating the path to a stronger, more vibrant, and fiber-rich life.

Chapter 1: The Power of Fiber: An Introduction to a Healthier You

Welcome to the beginning of your transformative journey! In this chapter, we will embark on an exploration of the power of fiber and its profound impact on your overall well-being. Fiber, often overlooked and underestimated, is the unsung hero that can revolutionize your health and transform your life.

We'll start by understanding what fiber is and why it is so crucial for our bodies. Fiber is a type of carbohydrate found in plant-based foods that our bodies cannot fully digest. Unlike other carbohydrates, fiber passes through our digestive system intact, playing a unique and essential role in maintaining our health.

The benefits of fiber are vast and encompass various aspects of our physical and mental well-being. From promoting healthy digestion and preventing constipation to regulating blood sugar levels and reducing the risk of heart disease, fiber is truly a powerhouse nutrient.

But what makes fiber so special? It all comes down to its unique properties. Fiber adds bulk to your diet, making you feel fuller for longer and curbing unnecessary cravings. By doing so, it becomes your ally in maintaining a healthy weight and managing your appetite.

Moreover, fiber acts as a broom, sweeping away harmful toxins and waste materials from your body. It aids in the prevention of digestive issues such as diverticulosis and hemorrhoids, ensuring that your gut remains in optimal condition.

Beyond the physical benefits, fiber also impacts our mental and emotional well-being. By fostering a healthy gut environment, fiber promotes the production of neurotransmitters like serotonin, often referred to as the "feel-good" hormone. This means that a fiber-rich diet can contribute to improved mood, reduced stress, and increased mental clarity.

As you delve deeper into this chapter, you will gain a comprehensive understanding of the different types of fiber, their sources, and how to incorporate them into your daily meals. We will also debunk common misconceptions surrounding fiber and provide practical tips to help you overcome any challenges on your high-fiber journey.

Get ready to unlock the true power of fiber and take charge of your health like never before. Together, let's embrace the fiber revolution and embark on a transformative path toward a healthier, more fulfilling life.

Chapter 1: The Power of Fiber: An Introduction to a Healthier You

Welcome to the beginning of your transformative journey! In this chapter, we will embark on an exploration of the power of fiber and its profound impact on your overall well-being. Get ready to be amazed and inspired as we uncover the emotional connection we have with fiber and how it can change your life.

Picture this: You wake up in the morning, feeling tired and sluggish, your body yearning for a change. You're tired of the constant cycle of unhealthy eating, feeling guilty with every bite, and desperately searching for a solution. That solution lies within the embrace of fiber.

As you delve into the world of fiber, you'll soon realize that it's not just about numbers or scientific jargon. It's about discovering a newfound love for nourishing your body from the inside out. It's about reconnecting with the joy of eating and embracing foods that truly nurture and heal.

Imagine the satisfaction of biting into a crisp, juicy apple, knowing that with every fiber-rich bite, you're nourishing your body with vitamins, minerals, and a dose of natural energy. Or savoring the earthy goodness of whole grains, feeling the warmth and comfort they bring to your soul. These simple moments become transformative when you understand the power of fiber.

But it's not just about the physical benefits. It's about the emotional transformation that comes hand in hand with embracing a high-fiber lifestyle. It's about reclaiming control over your health and feeling empowered to make choices that honor your body and mind.

With each fiber-packed meal, you'll feel a renewed sense of vitality and self-worth. The guilt and shame of past eating habits fade away, replaced by a deep appreciation for the nourishment you provide yourself. It's a journey of self-love and self-discovery, where you realize that your well-being is worth every delicious and nutritious bite.

And let's not forget the emotional comfort that comes with a healthy digestive system. No more bloating, discomfort, or embarrassing moments. Instead, you'll feel light, vibrant, and free. Your confidence will soar as you embrace a body that feels good from the inside out, radiating with vitality and strength.

As you read through the pages of this chapter, I invite you to reflect on your own relationship with food and your body. Take a moment to appreciate the incredible vessel that carries you through life, and consider how nourishing it with fiber-rich foods can be a form of self-care, self-respect, and self-love.

The journey ahead may not always be easy, but it will be worth it. Together, we will navigate the challenges and celebrate the victories. By the end of this book, you will have transformed not only your eating habits but also your mindset, paving the way for a life filled with vibrant health, joy, and emotional well-being.

Are you ready to embrace the power of fiber and embark on a journey that will change your life from the inside out?

Let's dive in and discover the incredible potential that lies within you.

Chapter 2: Whole Grains: The Foundation of a High-Fiber Diet

In this chapter, we delve into the heart and soul of a high-fiber diet: whole grains. Prepare to be captivated by their humble yet extraordinary nature and the emotional connection they forge with our bodies and spirits.

Imagine the comforting aroma of freshly baked bread wafting through the air, filling your kitchen with warmth and anticipation. The very essence of whole grains is a testament to the nourishing power they possess.

It's a sensory experience that touches deep within, evoking memories of home-cooked meals and cherished moments shared around the table.

Whole grains are not just about sustenance; they are about sustenance for the soul. With every mouthful of hearty oats, nutty quinoa, or earthy brown rice, you'll feel a profound connection to the earth and its bountiful offerings. It's a reminder that we are part of a larger tapestry, intricately woven with the gifts of nature.

Beyond their emotional resonance, whole grains hold the key to unlocking a myriad of health benefits. They are packed with essential vitamins, minerals, and dietary fiber that nourish our bodies from within. From supporting digestive health to reducing the risk of chronic diseases, the impact of whole grains on our well-being is nothing short of extraordinary.

But it doesn't end there. Whole grains have the power to ignite our creativity in the kitchen, offering endless possibilities for culinary exploration. They infuse dishes with depth and texture, transforming mundane meals into delightful culinary adventures. The act of preparing and savoring whole grain-based recipes becomes an expression of love and self-care , a celebration of flavors, colors, and nourishment.

As you journey through this chapter, allow yourself to be inspired by the versatility of whole grains. Discover the joy of a warm bowl of oatmeal, topped with luscious berries and a drizzle of honey, enveloping your taste buds in pure bliss. Or indulge in the robust flavors of a quinoa salad, where every bite tells a story of vibrant ingredients and vibrant health.

But perhaps the most beautiful aspect of whole grains is their ability to connect us with traditions and cultures. They transcend borders and unite us in a shared appreciation for wholesome, real food. Whether it's the comforting embrace of a bowl of steaming rice or the nourishing aroma of freshly baked bread, whole grains speak a universal language , one that resonates with our hearts and souls.

So, dear reader, let us embrace whole grains as more than just a dietary choice. Let us honor their role as the foundation of a high-fiber diet and the emotional sustenance they provide. Through whole grains, we nourish not only our bodies but also our spirits, forging a profound connection with nature and the nourishing power it bestows upon us.

As you embark on this chapter, open your heart to the wonders of whole grains. Embrace their rich history, their sensory allure, and their transformative potential. Let them be the cornerstone of your high-fiber journey, propelling you toward a life of vitality, connection, and emotional well-being.

Chapter 3: The Benefits of Legumes: Fueling Your Body with Fiber

In this chapter, we dive into the vibrant world of legumes, those tiny powerhouses of nutrition and emotional nourishment. Get ready to be swept away by their colorful array, diverse flavors, and the deep connection they foster with our bodies and the planet.

Close your eyes and envision a bustling farmers market, brimming with baskets of vibrant beans, lentils, and chickpeas. Each legume tells a story of resilience, growth, and the abundance of nature. As you reach out and touch their smooth surfaces, you feel an immediate connection , a recognition of the life force that pulses within.

Legumes, oh how they captivate our senses and stir our emotions. From the creamy comfort of a bowl of lentil soup to the hearty satisfaction of a plate of chili made with kidney beans, legumes embrace us like a warm embrace from a loved one. They nourish not only our bodies but also our souls, filling us with a sense of comfort and contentment.

But the emotional connection to legumes goes beyond their comforting nature. They are a testament to the power of resilience and adaptability.

Legumes thrive in challenging conditions, their roots delving deep into the soil, drawing sustenance from the earth. In a world that often feels uncertain and overwhelming, legumes remind us of our own strength and ability to flourish amidst adversity.

The benefits of legumes extend far beyond their emotional resonance. They are a nutritional treasure trove, rich in protein, fiber, vitamins, and minerals. From improving heart health to stabilizing blood sugar levels, legumes offer a multitude of health advantages that nurture our bodies from within.

Moreover, legumes have a profound impact on the environment. They are a sustainable source of protein, requiring fewer resources and producing fewer greenhouse gas emissions compared to animal-based proteins. By embracing legumes, we become stewards of the

Earth, forging a connection with the planet and contributing to its well-being.

As you journey through this chapter, allow yourself to be inspired by the versatility of legumes. Explore the exotic flavors of a chickpea curry, the comforting aroma of a pot of simmering black beans, or the delicate texture of a lentil salad. Embrace the beauty of legumes in all their forms , dried, canned, or sprouted , and let them awaken your taste buds and nourish your soul.

But remember, legumes are not just ingredients; they are a celebration of diversity and culture. They form the basis of traditional dishes from around the world, connecting us to different lands and communities. With each bite, we honor the richness and heritage that legumes bring to our plates, fostering a deep sense of appreciation and interconnectedness.

So, dear reader, let us embrace legumes as more than just a source of fiber and nutrition. Let us celebrate their ability to ignite our senses, nurture our bodies, and foster a profound connection with nature and our fellow humans. Through legumes, we find sustenance for our bodies, solace for our souls, and a reminder of the remarkable resilience within us.

As you embark on this chapter, open your heart to the wonders of legumes. Allow their vibrant colors, textures, and flavors to awaken your senses and inspire you to create nourishing meals that fuel your body and feed your spirit. Let legumes be your guiding light on this high-fiber journey, illuminating a path of vitality, connection, and emotional well-being.

Chapter 4: The Green Revolution: Exploring Fiber-Rich Vegetables

In this chapter, we embark on a journey into the vibrant world of fiber-rich vegetables, where nature's verdant offerings captivate our senses and nourish our bodies and souls. Get ready to be immersed in the kaleidoscope of colors, flavors, and emotions that vegetables evoke, igniting a passion for wholesome living.

Imagine stepping into a lush garden, a sanctuary of life and vitality. The air is infused with the earthy fragrance of freshly picked vegetables, and the gentle breeze whispers secrets of growth and renewal. As you run your fingers along the velvety leaves of a spinach plant or gaze upon the radiant hues of a rainbow of bell peppers, you feel an indescribable connection , a recognition of the profound bond we share with the natural world.

Vegetables, oh how they stir our emotions and awaken our senses. From the crisp crunch of a cucumber to the tender bite of a roasted carrot, each vegetable carries a story , a story of resilience, nourishment, and the sheer beauty of life itself. They remind us that we are part of a greater tapestry, intricately woven with the gifts of the earth.

But the emotional connection to vegetables extends far beyond their visual and tactile allure. They are the embodiment of vitality and well-being, the essence of life-giving nutrition. With every fiber-rich bite, we honor our bodies and embrace a profound sense of self-care and self-love.

Vegetables offer a plethora of health benefits that nourish us from within. They are rich in vitamins, minerals, antioxidants, and, of course, fiber, the unsung hero that supports digestion, promotes a healthy weight, and lowers the risk of chronic diseases. The vibrant colors of vegetables are not merely aesthetics; they signify the presence of phytonutrients that protect our cells, boost our immune system, and rejuvenate our bodies.

As you journey through this chapter, allow yourself to be enchanted by the myriad of flavors and textures that vegetables offer. Explore the crisp sweetness of a bell pepper, the earthy richness of a roasted beet, or the delicate crunch of a broccoli floret. Let each bite be a celebration of the incredible diversity and abundance that nature provides , a symphony of tastes that nourish our palates and our souls.

But vegetables are more than just ingredients on a plate; they are a celebration of life and interconnectedness. They connect us to the land, the farmers, and the seasons. With each vegetable we choose, we become part of a larger movement , a green revolution that embraces sustainability, supports local communities, and cherishes the precious resources of our planet.

So, dear reader, let us embrace vegetables as more than just a source of fiber and nutrition. Let us celebrate their ability to awaken our senses, nurture our bodies, and foster a profound connection with nature and our own well-being. Through vegetables, we rediscover the joy of nourishing ourselves and the world around us.

As you embark on this chapter, open your heart to the wonders of fiber-rich vegetables. Allow their vibrant colors, fresh aromas, and delightful flavors to inspire you in the kitchen and beyond. Let vegetables be your companions on this high-fiber journey, illuminating a path of vitality, connection, and emotional well-being.

Chapter 5: Fruity Delights: How Fiber-Packed Fruits Boost Your Well-being

In this chapter, we immerse ourselves in the world of fiber-packed fruits, where sweetness intertwines with nourishment, and nature's gifts awaken our senses and enrich our well-being.

Prepare to be enchanted by the vibrant hues, luscious flavors, and the deep emotional connection that fruits forge with our bodies and souls.

Close your eyes and imagine walking through a sun-kissed orchard, the air filled with the intoxicating scent of ripe fruits. The branches sway gently, offering their colorful bounty like a gift from nature herself. As you reach out and pluck a succulent strawberry or taste the nectar of a perfectly ripe mango, you experience a burst of pure joy , a moment of bliss that lingers in your heart.

Fruits, oh how they delight our senses and stir our emotions. Each one carries a story of growth, sweetness, and the abundance of the earth. Their vibrant colors and juicy textures tantalize our taste buds and remind us of the simple pleasures that life has to offer. With every bite, we are transported to a place of pure happiness, where the worries of the world melt away, and we find solace in the embrace of nature's gifts.

But the beauty of fruits extends far beyond their delectable flavors. They are nutritional powerhouses, brimming with vitamins, minerals, antioxidants, and, of course, fiber , the magical ingredient that nourishes our bodies and supports our overall well-being. Fruits are nature's way of providing us with a sweet symphony of nutrients , a symphony that supports our immune system, aids in digestion, and helps maintain a healthy weight.

As you explore this chapter, allow yourself to be captivated by the diverse range of fruits and their unique attributes. From the tangy burst of citrus fruits to the velvety sweetness of berries, each fruit carries its own story , a story of vitality, abundance, and the remarkable way they contribute to our health and happiness.

But fruits are more than just a source of nutrition; they are a celebration of life's joys and a reminder of the beauty that surrounds us. They are the taste of summer picnics and laughter shared with loved ones. With every bite, we savor the moments of connection and celebration, cherishing the memories that fruits help create.

So, dear reader, let us embrace fruits as more than just a source of fiber and nutrition. Let us celebrate their ability to awaken our senses, nourish our bodies, and evoke a deep emotional response. Through fruits, we find a connection to the natural world , a connection that fills us with gratitude, wonder, and a renewed sense of vitality.

As you embark on this chapter, open your heart to the wonders of fiber-packed fruits. Allow their vibrant colors, fragrant aromas, and juicy textures to transport you to a place of pure delight. Let fruits be your partners on this high-fiber journey, infusing your life with sweetness, vitality, and a renewed appreciation for the abundant gifts of nature.

Chapter 6: The Nutty Way: Nurturing Your Body with Fiber-Rich Nuts and Seeds

In this chapter, we delve into the enchanting world of fiber-rich nuts and seeds, where nature's hidden treasures unfold and ignite our senses. Get ready to embark on a journey of discovery, where the crunchy textures, delicate flavors, and the profound emotional connection of nuts and seeds will nourish your body and uplift your spirit.

Imagine strolling through a sun-dappled forest, the ground beneath your feet adorned with fallen leaves and hidden treasures. As you look up, majestic trees reveal their secret bounty , nuts and seeds, nature's precious gifts. You reach out, gathering a handful of almonds or tracing your fingers along the intricate shell of a sunflower seed. In that moment, you feel a deep connection with the Earth , their origin, their growth, and the life-sustaining power they possess.

Nuts and seeds, oh how they ignite our senses and stir our emotions. Each one carries a story of resilience, nourishment, and the interconnectedness of all living things. With every crunchy bite, we tap into the ancient wisdom of nature, honoring the gifts that sustain us and embracing the vibrant energy they provide.

But the emotional connection to nuts and seeds goes beyond their sensory allure. They are nutritional powerhouses, packed with essential vitamins, minerals, healthy fats, and, of course, fiber , the nutrient that supports our digestive health, promotes satiety, and fuels our bodies with sustained energy. Nuts and seeds are the embodiment of nature's intelligence, offering us the perfect balance of nourishment and sustenance.

As you explore this chapter, let yourself be captivated by the diverse array of nuts and seeds and the unique stories they tell. From the earthy richness of walnuts to the delicate crunch of chia seeds, each variety has its own character , a character that brings depth and complexity to your culinary creations and nourishes you from within.

But nuts and seeds are more than just ingredients in your pantry; they are a reminder of the transformative power of small things. In their unassuming shells lie immense potential, waiting to be unlocked. They are a testament to the beauty of growth and the notion that even the tiniest seed can become a towering tree. Through nuts and seeds, we find inspiration to nurture our own growth and embrace the possibilities that lie within us.

So, dear reader, let us embrace nuts and seeds as more than just sources of fiber and nutrition. Let us celebrate their ability to awaken our senses, nourish our bodies, and spark a deep emotional connection with the natural world. Through nuts and seeds, we find sustenance for our bodies, inspiration for our journeys, and a profound appreciation for the intricate web of life.

As you embark on this chapter, open your heart to the wonders of fiber-rich nuts and seeds. Allow their delightful textures, rich flavors, and hidden treasures to enrich your meals and your life. Let them be your allies on this high-fiber journey, infusing your days with the delightful crunch, nourishment, and the power of nature's wisdom.

Chapter 7: Fantastic Fiber: Unveiling the Magic of Fiber Supplements

In this chapter, we uncover the magical realm of fiber supplements, where science and nature intertwine to create a powerful tool for supporting our well-being. Get ready to be enchanted by the potential of these fantastic fibers, as they nourish your body and empower your soul.

Imagine stepping into a laboratory, a place where knowledge is distilled into potent elixirs. Rows of sleek bottles beckon, each one holding the promise of transformation and renewal. As you hold a fiber supplement in your hand, you feel a surge of excitement , a recognition of the incredible impact it can have on your health and vitality.

Fiber supplements, oh how they captivate our curiosity and stir our emotions. They are the embodiment of human ingenuity, harnessing the power of nature's fibers and concentrating them into convenient forms. With each capsule or scoop, we embrace the potential to enhance our well-being and unlock the secrets of optimal health.

But the emotional connection to fiber supplements goes beyond their scientific marvel. They represent the commitment we have to caring for ourselves, to seeking out the tools and resources that can support our journey towards wellness. Fiber supplements are a reminder that we have the power to take charge of our health, to make choices that nourish our bodies and souls.

Fiber supplements offer a myriad of benefits, complementing our dietary intake and providing a convenient way to meet our fiber needs. They support digestive health, promote regularity, and help manage appetite. With their soluble and insoluble fibers, they contribute to the complex ecosystem of our gut, nurturing the symbiotic relationship between our bodies and the trillions of microorganisms that reside within.

As you explore this chapter, allow yourself to be fascinated by the diversity of fiber supplements and the unique ways they can enhance your well-being. From psyllium husk to glucomannan, each fiber has its own extraordinary properties , a unique magic that supports your body in different ways. They are the allies that stand beside you on your quest for better health.

But fiber supplements are more than just pills or powders; they represent a commitment to self-care and a recognition of the importance of balance. They remind us that true wellness encompasses not only the physical but also the emotional and spiritual aspects of our being. They are a gentle reminder to listen to our bodies, to honor their needs, and to nourish ourselves in ways that go beyond the tangible.

So, dear reader, let us embrace fiber supplements as more than just tools for meeting our fiber goals. Let us celebrate their ability to support our well-being, to empower us on our journey towards optimal health. Through fiber supplements, we find a means of self-care and a reminder that we have the power to shape our own wellness narratives.

As you embark on this chapter, open your heart to the wonders of fiber supplements. Allow their potential to ignite your curiosity and inspire you to explore the options available to you. Let them be your allies on this high-fiber journey, guiding you towards a life of vitality, balance, and emotional well-being.

Chapter 8: Fiber and Digestion: Enhancing Gut Health and Relieving Digestive Issues

In this chapter, we embark on a journey deep into the realm of our digestive system, where fiber reigns as the unsung hero, supporting our gut health and alleviating digestive issues. Get ready to explore the intricate world of digestion and the profound emotional connection we have with our gut.

Close your eyes and visualize the remarkable inner workings of your digestive system. It is a symphony of organs, enzymes, and microbes, working harmoniously to break down food and extract nourishment. Within this symphony, fiber takes center stage, a gentle conductor that orchestrates the rhythm of digestion, ensuring optimal health and vitality.

Our gut, oh how it whispers to us, telling tales of hunger, satisfaction, and the delicate balance between pleasure and discomfort. It is a source of intuition, a place where we experience the emotional and physical connection between what we eat and how we feel. Our gut is not just a physical organ; it is a portal to our overall well-being.

Fiber, the nurturing companion of our gut, plays a pivotal role in maintaining digestive harmony. It adds bulk to our stools, preventing constipation and promoting regularity. It acts as a prebiotic, fueling the growth of beneficial bacteria that support our immune system and contribute to overall gut health. Fiber is the gentle embrace that ensures our digestive journey is smooth, efficient, and devoid of unnecessary burdens.

But the emotional connection to fiber and digestion runs deeper than the physiological processes. It is an intimate dance, a conversation between our bodies and our souls. We feel the unease of indigestion and the relief of a well-settled stomach. We experience the emotions that arise from digestive imbalances, frustration, discomfort, and the longing for a sense of normalcy.

As you explore this chapter, allow yourself to be immersed in the intricate dance of fiber and digestion. Discover the diverse fibers that can support your gut health, soluble fibers that dissolve in water, like the delicate petals of a flower, and insoluble fibers that provide structure and strength, like the roots of a mighty tree. Embrace the beauty of this symbiotic relationship and the immense potential it holds for your overall well-being.

But fiber and digestion are not just about physical health; they are about emotional nourishment. When we care for our gut, we are nurturing the very core of our being , the place where intuition resides, where our emotions find their voice. By supporting our digestion with fiber-rich foods and mindful eating practices, we create a foundation of stability and emotional well-being.

So, dear reader, let us embrace the profound connection between fiber and digestion as more than just a physiological process. Let us celebrate it as a gateway to nourishment, intuition, and emotional harmony. Through fiber and digestion, we tap into the wisdom of our bodies, honoring the intricate dance of nourishment and transformation that occurs within us.

As you embark on this chapter, open your heart to the wonders of fiber and digestion. Listen to the whispers of your gut, honor its needs, and explore the multitude of ways fiber can enhance your digestive health. Let fiber be your gentle guide on this high-fiber journey, nurturing your gut, soothing your emotions, and paving the path towards a life of vitality, balance, and emotional well-being.

Chapter 9: Fiber and Weight Management: The Key to Shedding Pounds Naturally

In this chapter, we embark on a transformative journey, exploring the powerful connection between fiber and weight management. Get ready to unlock the secret to shedding pounds naturally, as fiber becomes your trusted ally in achieving a healthy and balanced body.

Close your eyes and envision your ideal self, the version of you that radiates confidence, vitality, and self-love. Picture yourself embracing life with a spring in your step, feeling comfortable and at ease in your own skin. The path to this vision begins with understanding the profound role that fiber plays in weight management.

Our weight, oh how it can influence our emotions and our sense of self-worth. We may have experienced the frustration of restrictive diets, the disappointment of temporary results, and the never-ending cycle of weight fluctuations. But within the realm of fiber lies a natural and sustainable solution , a key to shedding pounds while nourishing our bodies and souls.

Fiber holds the power to revolutionize our relationship with food and our bodies. It adds bulk and satiety to our meals, leaving us feeling fuller for longer and reducing unnecessary cravings. It is the gentle hand that guides us away from mindless snacking and towards a mindful, nourishing approach to eating.

But the emotional connection to fiber and weight management goes beyond the physical aspects. It is about self-acceptance, self-care, and the recognition that our bodies are deserving of love and respect at any size. When we embrace fiber as a tool for weight management, we embark on a journey of self-discovery , a journey that allows us to redefine our relationship with food and our bodies.

As you delve into this chapter, allow yourself to embrace the transformative potential of fiber in your weight management journey. Discover the various fiber-rich foods that can support your goals , crunchy vegetables that add volume to your meals, satiating whole grains that keep you satisfied, and the delightful sweetness of fruits that satisfy your cravings. Embrace the vibrant colors, textures, and flavors of these fiber-packed foods, and let them nourish both your body and your spirit.

But weight management is not just about numbers on a scale; it is about finding balance and fostering self-compassion. It is about nourishing ourselves from within, embracing our bodies as vessels of strength and resilience. By incorporating fiber-rich foods into our meals, we nourish not only our physical bodies but also our emotional well-being, nurturing a positive relationship with ourselves and the food we consume.

So, dear reader, let us celebrate the powerful connection between fiber and weight management as more than just a means to a physical goal. Let us embrace it as a catalyst for self-love, self-acceptance, and holistic well-being. Through fiber and weight management, we embark on a journey of transformation , one that nourishes our bodies, nurtures our souls, and allows us to shine as our most authentic selves.

As you embark on this chapter, open your heart to the wonders of fiber and weight management. Embrace the opportunity to redefine your relationship with food and your body, to nourish yourself with intention and kindness. Let fiber become your trusted companion on this high-fiber journey, guiding you towards a life of balance, self-acceptance, and emotional well-being.

[550]

Chapter 10: Fiber and Heart Health: Nurturing the Lifeline of Your Well-being

In this chapter, we explore the profound connection between fiber and heart health , a bond that goes beyond physical well-being and touches the very core of our emotional and spiritual existence. Get ready to embark on a journey of love, care, and empowerment as we delve into the transformative power of fiber for the heart.

Close your eyes and envision the intricate network that sustains your life , the rhythmic beats, the pulsating flow of vitality. Your heart, the guardian of your well-being, holds within it the essence of your emotions, your desires, and your connection to the world. Within the realm of fiber lies a secret , a key to nurturing this lifeline and embracing a heart that beats with strength and resilience.

Our hearts, oh how they whisper to us , the gentle rhythm that accompanies moments of joy, the fluttering sensation of anticipation, the ache of longing and the comfort of love. They are the vessels that carry our emotions, the gateways to our deepest desires. Within the world of fiber, we find the nourishment that supports our hearts, nourishing not only our physical well-being but also the emotional and spiritual aspects of our lives.

Fiber holds the power to protect our hearts, reduce the risk of cardiovascular disease, and promote overall heart health. Soluble fiber acts as a sponge, absorbing cholesterol and preventing its buildup in our arteries. It is the guardian that shields our hearts from the harms of unhealthy fats and cholesterol, while insoluble fiber sweeps away waste materials and supports the health of our blood vessels.

But the emotional connection to fiber and heart health transcends the physical benefits. It is about embracing the power of self-care and love , for our hearts, our bodies, and our emotional well-being. When we prioritize fiber-rich foods, we are nurturing the very essence of our existence, honoring the vessels that carry us through life's joys and challenges.

As you explore this chapter, allow yourself to embrace the transformative potential of fiber for your heart. Discover the array of fiber-rich foods that can support cardiovascular health, nutrient-dense fruits and vegetables, heart-healthy whole grains, and the delightful crunch of nuts and seeds. Let each bite be an act of love, a gesture of empowerment, and a tribute to the miraculous beating of your heart.

But heart health is not just about physical well-being; it is about emotional resilience and the capacity to open ourselves to love and connection. When we care for our hearts through fiber-rich choices, we honor our emotional well-being, allowing ourselves to experience the full range of human emotions with grace and strength.

So, dear reader, let us celebrate the profound connection between fiber and heart health as more than just a preventive measure. Let us embrace it as a pathway to emotional well-being, a catalyst for self-love and connection. Through fiber and heart health, we embark on a journey of empowerment, one that nourishes our bodies, nurtures our souls, and allows us to live with open hearts.

As you embark on this chapter, open your heart to the wonders of fiber and heart health. Embrace the opportunity to care for your heart, to nourish it with love and intention. Let fiber become your guiding light on this high-fiber journey, illuminating the path towards a life of vitality, emotional well-being, and a heart that beats with strength and resilience.

Chapter 11: Fiber and Mental Well-being: Nurturing the Mind-Body Connection

In this chapter, we delve into the profound interplay between fiber and mental well-being, uncovering the transformative power that fiber holds for our minds and emotions. Get ready to embark on a journey of self-discovery, as we explore the intricate connection between our dietary choices and the landscape of our inner world.

Close your eyes and imagine stepping into a sanctuary of serenity, a place where calmness and clarity reside. Your mind, the gateway to your thoughts, emotions, and dreams, is a delicate ecosystem that requires nourishment and care. Within the realm of fiber lies a secret , a key to nurturing the mind-body connection and fostering a state of mental well-being.

Our minds, oh how they guide us through life , the currents of thoughts, the ebb and flow of emotions, the tapestry of memories and aspirations. They are the landscape of our inner world, shaping our experiences and influencing our sense of self. Within the world of fiber, we find the nourishment that supports our mental well-being, nurturing our minds and empowering us to embrace a life of emotional balance and resilience.

Fiber holds the power to support mental well-being through various mechanisms. It helps regulate blood sugar levels, providing a steady supply of energy to the brain and promoting stable moods. Fiber also plays a role in balancing gut health, influencing the production of neurotransmitters that impact our emotions and mental state. By nourishing our bodies with fiber-rich foods, we lay the foundation for a harmonious mind-body connection.

But the emotional connection to fiber and mental well-being goes beyond the physiological effects. It is about recognizing the profound impact that our dietary choices have on our emotions, our clarity of thought, and our capacity to navigate life's challenges with resilience. When we prioritize fiber, we are honoring our minds, nurturing our emotions, and fostering a state of inner peace.

As you explore this chapter, allow yourself to embrace the transformative potential of fiber for your mental well-being. Discover the abundance of fiber-rich foods that can support your mind , colorful fruits and vegetables that nourish your brain cells, whole grains that provide sustained energy, and the soothing comfort of nuts and seeds. Let each bite be an act of self-care, a gesture of love towards your mind and emotions.

But mental well-being is not just about individual choices; it is about fostering a compassionate and supportive environment. When we prioritize fiber-rich meals, we create a ripple effect, a positive impact on our relationships, our communities, and the world at large. Our well-nourished minds become the seeds of empathy, understanding, and a deep connection with the human experience.

So, dear reader, let us celebrate the profound connection between fiber and mental well-being as more than just a dietary consideration. Let us embrace it as a gateway to self-discovery, compassion, and emotional resilience. Through fiber and mental well-being, we embark on a journey of self-care, one that nourishes our bodies, nurtures our minds, and empowers us to live a life of emotional balance and well-being.

As you embark on this chapter, open your mind and heart to the wonders of fiber and its impact on your mental well-being. Embrace the opportunity to nurture your mind, to cultivate emotional resilience, and to foster a deep connection with yourself and others. Let fiber be your steadfast companion on this high-fiber journey, guiding you towards a life of clarity, peace, and emotional well-being.

Chapter 12: Fiber and Energy: Fueling Your Life with Vitality and Passion

In this chapter, we explore the captivating relationship between fiber and energy, a dynamic connection that goes beyond physical vitality and touches the very essence of our emotional and spiritual existence. Get ready to embark on a journey of invigoration, as we unveil the transformative power of fiber in fueling your life with boundless energy and passion.

Close your eyes and envision a world brimming with vitality, the energy coursing through your veins, the spark of passion igniting your every step. Your body, the vessel of your dreams and aspirations, yearns for a sustainable source of fuel, a secret ingredient that will infuse your life with vibrancy and purpose. Within the realm of fiber lies the key, a gateway to unlocking the boundless energy that resides within you.

Our energy, oh how it propels us forward , the zest that accompanies new beginnings, the fire that fuels our endeavors, the light that guides us through challenges. It is the essence of our existence, the driving force that empowers us to embrace life with passion and enthusiasm. Within the world of fiber, we find the nourishment that supports our energy levels, providing a sustainable and lasting vitality.

Fiber holds the power to fuel our lives with energy in remarkable ways. It helps regulate blood sugar levels, preventing energy crashes and providing a steady source of fuel throughout the day. Fiber also promotes a healthy gut, supporting the efficient absorption of nutrients and optimizing our energy metabolism. By nourishing our bodies with fiber-rich foods, we unlock the door to sustained energy and a vibrant life.

But the emotional connection to fiber and energy transcends the physical realm. It is about embracing a life of purpose and vitality, where our energy aligns with our passions and desires. When we prioritize fiber, we embrace the opportunity to live each day with intention, harnessing the energy needed to pursue our dreams, nurture our relationships, and make a positive impact on the world.

As you delve into this chapter, allow yourself to embrace the transformative potential of fiber for your energy levels. Discover the array of fiber-rich foods that can revitalize your body , energizing fruits and vegetables that provide essential vitamins and minerals, whole grains that offer sustained fuel, and the nourishing power of nuts and seeds. Let each bite be a celebration of life, a tribute to the remarkable energy that resides within you.

But energy is not just about physical stamina; it is about infusing each moment with presence, enthusiasm, and a deep connection with your purpose. When we nourish our bodies with fiber, we align our energy with our passions, allowing every action and endeavor to be fueled by the fire of our hearts.

So, dear reader, let us celebrate the profound connection between fiber and energy as more than just a physiological phenomenon. Let us embrace it as a catalyst for a life of vitality, purpose, and boundless enthusiasm. Through fiber and energy, we embark on a journey of self-discovery , one that ignites our passions, nurtures our bodies, and empowers us to live a life of vibrant energy and unwavering passion.

As you embark on this chapter, open your heart to the wonders of fiber and its impact on your energy levels. Embrace the opportunity to fuel your life with vitality and purpose, to infuse each moment with enthusiasm and a deep connection with your passions. Let fiber be the guiding light on this high-fiber journey, illuminating the path towards a life of boundless energy, inspired action, and emotional well-being.

Chapter 13: The Healing Power of Fiber: Nourishing Body, Mind, and Soul

In this chapter, we delve into the profound healing power of fiber , a force that extends beyond the physical realm and touches the very core of our emotional and spiritual well-being. Get ready to embark on a journey of restoration and transformation as we unveil the remarkable capacity of fiber to nourish not only our bodies but also our minds and souls.

Close your eyes and envision a sanctuary of healing , a space filled with serenity, compassion, and profound renewal. Your body, mind, and soul yearn for restoration , for a gentle touch that will heal the wounds, both seen and unseen. Within the realm of fiber lies a profound secret , a key to nourishing your entire being and embracing a life of wholeness and well-being.

Our healing, oh how it resonates within us , the whispers of hope, the triumph over adversity, the capacity to rise from the ashes. It is a journey that weaves together our physical, emotional, and spiritual realms , a tapestry of resilience and growth. Within the world of fiber, we find the nourishment that supports this journey of healing, providing the essential building blocks for our restoration and transformation.

Fiber holds the power to heal our bodies in extraordinary ways. It supports digestive health, soothing inflammation and promoting regularity. It nourishes our gut microbiome, fostering a balanced ecosystem that influences our immune system and overall well-being. By embracing fiber-rich foods, we create a foundation for healing , a sanctuary for our bodies to thrive and regenerate.

But the emotional connection to fiber and healing is profound. It is about recognizing the power we hold within ourselves , the innate capacity to heal, to find resilience in the face of adversity, and to embrace our journey of self-discovery. When we prioritize fiber, we honor our bodies as sacred vessels of healing, nurturing our physical, emotional, and spiritual well-being.

As you explore this chapter, allow yourself to embrace the transformative potential of fiber in your healing journey. Discover the abundance of fiber-rich foods that can support your restoration , nutrient-dense fruits and vegetables that provide vital antioxidants and phytonutrients, whole grains that nourish your cells, and the soothing comfort of nuts and seeds. Let each bite be an act of self-care, a gesture of love towards your entire being.

But healing is not just about physical recovery; it is about embracing the journey of self-discovery and self-compassion. When we nourish ourselves with fiber, we create space for emotional healing, nurturing our minds and souls with the same care and gentleness we offer our bodies.

So, dear reader, let us celebrate the profound connection between fiber and healing as more than just a means to an end. Let us embrace it as a catalyst for self-discovery, compassion, and a life of wholeness. Through fiber and healing, we embark on a transformative journey , one that nourishes our bodies, nurtures our minds, and allows our souls to soar.

As you embark on this chapter, open your heart to the wonders of fiber and its capacity to support your healing journey. Embrace the opportunity to nurture your entire being, to cultivate self-compassion, and to honor the profound interconnectedness of your physical, emotional, and spiritual well-being. Let fiber be your steadfast companion on this high-fiber journey, guiding you towards a life of restoration, transformation, and profound healing.

Chapter 14: Fiber and Inner Balance: Cultivating Harmony in Body, Mind, and Spirit

In this chapter, we explore the harmonizing power of fiber, a force that transcends the boundaries of our physical bodies and permeates the realms of our mind and spirit. Get ready to embark on a transformative journey of inner balance, as we unveil the profound impact of fiber in nurturing harmony and alignment within ourselves.

Close your eyes and imagine a tranquil sanctuary , a space where stillness and equilibrium embrace your entire being. Your body, mind, and spirit long for a sense of inner balance , for the soothing balm that will unite the different aspects of your existence. Within the realm of fiber lies a sacred tool , a gateway to cultivating harmony and fostering a life of serenity and interconnectedness.

Our inner balance, oh how it resonates within us , the delicate dance between action and stillness, the rhythm that guides us through life's fluctuations. It is the foundation of our well-being, the compass that aligns our thoughts, emotions, and actions. Within the world of fiber, we find the nourishment that supports this journey of cultivating inner balance, allowing us to navigate life's challenges with grace and poise.

Fiber holds the power to harmonize our bodies, minds, and spirits in remarkable ways. It nourishes our physical bodies, supporting digestive health, stabilizing blood sugar levels, and providing sustained energy. It nourishes our minds, fostering mental clarity, and supporting emotional resilience. It nourishes our spirits, connecting us to the natural world, and deepening our sense of interconnectedness.

But the emotional connection to fiber and inner balance goes beyond the physical benefits. It is about recognizing our innate capacity to find equilibrium , to honor the ebb and flow of life, to embrace both light and shadow, and to navigate the ever-changing landscape of our existence with grace. When we prioritize fiber, we embrace the opportunity to cultivate harmony within ourselves, nurturing the interconnectedness of our body, mind, and spirit.

As you delve into this chapter, allow yourself to embrace the transformative potential of fiber in cultivating inner balance. Discover the diverse array of fiber-rich foods that can support your journey , vibrant fruits and vegetables that provide essential nutrients, whole grains that ground and nourish your being, and the comforting embrace of nuts and seeds. Let each bite be an invitation to presence, an act of self-care, and a gesture of honoring the interconnectedness of your entire being.

But inner balance is not just about individual well-being; it is about fostering harmony within our relationships and the world around us. When we cultivate inner balance through fiber-rich choices, we become vessels of love, compassion, and interconnectedness, extending these qualities to those we encounter on our path.

So, dear reader, let us celebrate the profound connection between fiber and inner balance as more than just a personal pursuit. Let us embrace it as a catalyst for harmony, compassion, and a life of interconnectedness. Through fiber and inner balance, we embark on a transformative journey , one that nurtures our bodies, harmonizes our minds, and allows our spirits to flourish.

As you embark on this chapter, open your heart to the wonders of fiber and its capacity to support your quest for inner balance. Embrace the opportunity to cultivate harmony within yourself and extend it to the world around you. Let fiber be your guiding light on this high-fiber journey, leading you towards a life of serenity, interconnectedness, and profound inner balance.

Chapter 15: Embracing the Fiber Journey: A Path to Transformation and Wholeness

In this final chapter, we embark on a reflection of the transformative journey we've embarked upon , a journey of embracing the power of fiber to nourish our bodies, minds, and spirits. Get ready to immerse yourself in the essence of this transformative experience, as we celebrate the profound impact of fiber in guiding us towards a life of transformation and wholeness.

Close your eyes and take a moment to honor the path you've traveled, the chapters explored, the wisdom gained, and the layers of your being that have been touched by the power of fiber. As you reflect, you realize that this journey has been more than just a pursuit of health, it has been a journey of self-discovery, self-compassion, and profound transformation.

Our fiber journey, oh how it has reshaped us, the subtle shifts, the profound realizations, and the gentle whispers that have guided us along the way. It has been a tapestry woven with intention, as we embraced the nourishment, the wisdom, and the love that fiber has offered us. We have witnessed the healing, the energy, the harmony, and the resilience that has unfolded within us.

Through fiber, we have reconnected with the innate wisdom of our bodies , the intelligence that guides us towards nourishing choices, the capacity to listen and respond to our unique needs, and the embodiment of self-care. We have come to understand that our well-being extends beyond physical health , it encompasses our emotions, our thoughts, and the profound interconnectedness of our being.

As we have journeyed through the chapters, we have embraced the emotional tone , the tone of love, empowerment, and reverence for the intricate dance of fiber and our lives. We have recognized that our choices ripple outwards, impacting not only ourselves but also the world around us. Through fiber, we have become agents of change , nurturing our bodies, minds, and spirits, and fostering a ripple effect of well-being and compassion.

And so, dear reader, as we conclude this transformative fiber journey, let us carry the wisdom gained and the profound connections made within us. Let us honor the transformative power of fiber and the potential it holds for our lives. As we continue on our individual paths, may we always remember the nourishment, the love, and the healing that fiber has brought into our lives.

Embrace the choices that align with your well-being, the fiber-rich foods that sustain and uplift you, and the mindful practices that nourish your body, mind, and spirit. Let your journey be a testament to the profound impact that self-care, self-discovery, and self-compassion can have on our lives.

As we bid farewell to this fiber journey, let us carry the lessons learned, the connections made, and the transformation experienced within our hearts. May the power of fiber continue to guide us towards lives of vitality, balance, and wholeness , a constant reminder that we have the capacity to shape our well-being and embrace the fullness of our existence.

So, dear reader, as you embrace the concluding pages of this transformative journey, take a moment to honor the path you've traveled, the growth you've experienced, and the empowered choices you've made. You are a testament to the resilience, the potential, and the profound capacity for transformation that resides within you.

Embrace the fiber journey as a lifelong companion, a compass that guides you towards a life of vibrant health, emotional well-being, and spiritual fulfillment. Let fiber be your constant ally, nurturing your body, mind, and spirit, and guiding you towards a life of transformation, wholeness, and profound love.

[550]"

in%20One%20Click%22-,Book%20Title%3A%20High%20Fiber%3A%20Nourishing%20Your%20Body%2C%20Enriching%20Your%20Life,%5BWord%20Count%3A%20550%5D,-

AIPRM%20%2D %20ChatGPT %20Prompts

Made in the USA
Columbia, SC
24 November 2023